TIPS FOR LIVING HEALTHY: Plant-Based Diet for Beginners

Madison Sinclair

TABLE OF CONTENTS

INTRODUCTION

Ever tried following a plant-based diet? Going plant-based means eating solely soy products, salads, and other uninteresting foods for a lot of individuals. Yet nothing could be further from the truth than this. A plant-based diet is full of flavor, richness, and minerals. Simply described, plant-based diets are ways of eating that emphasize things like fruits, vegetables, nuts, seeds, legumes, and more that come from plants. Being able to design your own unique diet depending on your tastes is one of the best things about being plant-based. You can either go to a plant-based diet entirely and stop consuming any animal products, or you can continue consuming tiny amounts of animal products like dairy and eggs while concentrating mostly on plant sources.

Modes:

Instead, you can diversify your diet by discovering how truly delicious plant-based foods can be.

These days, prioritizing your health is of the essence. You want to be at the peak of your health in order to avoid illnesses. One of the best ways to do this is by improving your diet. You can do this by adding more plants to your plate. This book will help you out.

It's the perfect book for beginner to intermediate cooks who want to eat healthier foods. This book includes recipes for breakfast, lunch, dinner, snacks, smoothies, soups, and more. If you're looking for easy, delicious, simple, and inexpensive recipes to make, this is the cookbook for you!

To make things easy for you, the recipes here are neatly organized. They also use ingredients that you either have at home or are easy to get at the store. Each recipe includes the ingredients, steps, and even basic nutritional information. The latter can be very helpful if you want to achieve weight loss and other health goals. Going plant-bascd docsn't always mean becoming healthier.

Instead, you can broaden your dietary options by learning just how tasty plant-based foods can be.

These days, it's crucial to put your health first. To avoid sicknesses, you want to be in the best possible health. The greatest method to achieve this is through making dietary improvements. By include more plants on your meal, you can achieve this. You can get aid from this book.

It's the ideal cookbook for people who wish to consume healthier cuisine and are beginner to intermediate cooks. This book has recipes for smoothies, soups, breakfast, lunch, and dinner. This cookbook is for you if you're looking for economical, quick, delicious, and simple meals to prepare.

The recipes here are simplified for your convenience so nicely arranged. Additionally, they employ materials that you either already have at home or can easily purchase at a store. Every recipe contains a list of the components, the processes, and even some basic nutritional data. The latter is highly beneficial if you wish to lose weight and accomplish other health objectives. Going vegan doesn't always equate to being healthier.

I can attest to the many excellent advantages of a plant-based diet as someone who has successfully made the switch. I've gained more energy since switching to a plant-based diet, and I also feel fantastic! I also learned how very varied plant sources are. You can make incredibly delicious and nourishing dishes by combining various ingredients. They will leave you craving more.

I've experimented with cooking various plant-based foods for a while. I even experimented with meals from various cuisines. The beautiful thing about these recipes is that a lot of them are completely adaptable, so you can change up the ingredients to suit your tastes. I have compiled some of the best, most tasty dishes after experimenting with innumerable recipes to produce this recipe book. You will have a ton of recipes to test at home by the time this book is finished, meals that will help you achieve your health objectives.

Have you started salivating yet?

CHAPTER 1

A PLANT-BASED DIET IS WHAT?

There are so many different diets available nowadays. Each of these diets has certain guidelines and health objectives. The majority of the most popular diets, however, encourage the consumption of fresh, whole, and natural foods while minimizing the consumption of processed or packaged meals, as you'll find out if you try to look into the majority of them. Your general health will improve as a result of doing this because you'll be feeding your body the right foods. Simply because plant-based diets emphasize consuming full, healthy foods, you can reap the benefits of the healthiest diets by switching to one. You would concentrate on plant foods for such diets. It depends on you what kind of plant-based diet you would adopt.

The various types include:

.a semi-vegetarian or flexitarian diet that allows you to consume dairy and eggs. You could occasionally eat meat, poultry, fish, and seafood while following this diet.

.a diet that is primarily composed of fish, seafood, eggs, and dairy items. You wouldn't, however, cat any meat or poultry.

.a vegan diet consists entirely of plant foods and

excludes all animal products.

.a vegetarian or lacto-ovo vegetarian diet that forbids the consumption of meat, shellfish, poultry, or other animal products.

Going plant-based is fantastic because it gives you the freedom to choose what to include in your meals. You are not required to adhere to a schedule or abide by rigid regulations.

Why You Need to Cut Back On Processed and Animal-Based Products

You've probably heard time and time again that processed food is bad for you.

"Avoid preservatives; avoid processed foods"; however, no one ever really gives you any real or solid information on why you should avoid them and why they are dangerous. So let's break it down so that you can fully understand why you should avoid these culprits.

*They have huge addictive properties

As humans, we really have a strong tendency to be addicted to certain foods, but the fact is that it's not entirely our fault.

Practically all of the unhealthy eats we indulge in, from time to time, activate our brains dopamine neurotransmitter. This makes the brain feel "good" but only for a short period of time. This also creates an addiction tendency; that is why someone will always find themselves going back for another candy bar – even though they don't really need it. You can avoid all this by removing that stimulus altogether.

*They are loaded sugar and high fructose corn syrup Processed and animal-based products are loaded with sugars and high fructose.

Numerous studies are now confirming what many people already knew: that eating foods that have been genetically engineered causes intestinal inflammation, which makes it more difficult for the body to absorb nutrients.

One cannot overstate the importance of necessary nutrients for anything from fat accumulation and muscle loss.

*They include a ton of refined carbs.

Refined carbohydrates are abundant in processed foods and products made from animals. Yes, it is true that your body requires carbohydrates in order to function properly.

However, refining carbs removes the necessary elements, similar to how Whole grain content is removed during refinement. What's left of you After refinement, what are known as "empty" carbohydrates are produced. These may include a negatively affects your metabolism by increasing insulin and blood sugar levels.

*They contain a ton of artificial substances.

Your body perceives artificial compounds as foreign substances when you consume them. They essentially turn into an intrusion. Your body is unaccustomed to identifying Sucralose and other artificial sweeteners are examples. Your body then acts accordingly.

It decreases your resistance by inducing an immunological reaction, so you are susceptible to illnesses. Your body's concentration and energy are expended in,Otherwise, your immune system's efforts might be better spent elsewhere.

*They have ingredients that make your body feel overly rewarded.

This means that they contain ingredients like monosodium glutamate (MSG), high fructose corn syrup ingredients, and certain colours that have the potential to have addictive tendencies. Your body is stimulated so that you can benefit from it. For instance, many pre-packaged pastries include MSG. This encourages you to enjoy the taste by stimulating your taste buds. Just the way your brain interacts with your taste buds makes it psychological.

Veggie vs. Vegan Diet

People frequently confuse a vegan diet for a plant-based diet, or the other way around. Nevertheless, despite the similarities between the two diets, they are not exactly exact same So let's quickly deconstruct it.

Vegan

A vegan diet excludes anything made from animals.

This includes foods originating from animals, such as honey, as well as dairy, eggs, and meat.

A person who identifies as vegan incorporates this viewpoint into their daily activities. This means that they don't wear or advocate the wearing of clothing, footwear, accessories, shampoo, or cosmetics that contain materials derived from animals. Wool, beeswax, leather, gelatin, silk, and lanolin are a few examples here.

People who adopt a vegan lifestyle are frequently driven by a desire to take a position against animal abuse, unethical treatment of animals, and the promotion of animal rights.

Vegetarian Diet

On the other hand, a whole food plant-based diet is comparable to veganism in that it discourages the dietary consumption of goods derived from animals. Among them are dairy, beef, and eggs. In addition, unlike the vegan diet, the diet excludes processed foods, white flour, oils, and refined sugars. Making a diet of minimally processed to unprocessed fruits, vegetables, whole grains, nuts, seeds, and legumes is the objective here. Therefore, you won't be getting any Oreo cookies.

Followers of whole-food plant-based diets are frequently motivated by the health advantages it offers. It's a diet that doesn't focus much on calculating calories or calorie restriction macros, primarily focused on preventing and curing illness.

How to Start Eating Whole Foods from Plants

Many people, including some people working in the health and fitness industry, have the misconception that switching to a plant-based diet will instantly make you super healthy. There are several plant-based junk foods available, like non-dairy ice cream and frozen vegetable pizza, which, if regularly consumed, can seriously jeopardize your health goals. The only way to obtain health benefits is to commit to eating nutritious foods.On the other hand, you can stay motivated by eating these plant-based snacks. They ought to be eaten sparingly, in moderation, and in tiny amounts. There is a chapter in this book that is devoted to providing ideas for plant-based snacks you may make at home, as you will see in the later chapters. Here is how to begin a whole food plant-based recipe, without further ado.

Determine for Yourself What a Plant-Based Diet Means: The first stage will help you shift from your present diet outlook and is to decide how your plant-based diet will be structured. This is a very individual matter that differs from person to person. While some people decide they won't tolerate any animal products at all, others manage with sporadic small amounts of dairy or meat. You are ultimately in charge of deciding what and how your plant-based diet will be structured. The most crucial factor is that a sizable portion of your diet must consist of entire, plant-based meals.

Recognize the Food You Are Eating: Okay, now that you've mastered the decision-making process, your next task will require extensive analysis on your part. How do we interpret this? Well, if you're trying out a plant-based diet for the first time, you might be startled by how many goods, particularly packaged foods, include animal components. While shopping, you'll realize that you're cultivating the habit of reading labels. It turns out that many pre-packaged goods contain animal products, so you'll need to pay close attention to ingredient labels if you want to stick to just plant items for your new diet.

Find Updated Recipes for Your Favorite Dishes: You probably have a few go-to recipes that aren't entirely plant-based. The hardest aspect for most individuals is probably leaving all that behind. There is still a means for you to reach an accommodation, nevertheless. Think about the aspects of those meals that aren't plant-based that you enjoy. Consider things like flavor, texture, adaptability, and so on. Then, search for alternatives in a whole-foods plant-based diet that can replace the things you will be missing. Here are a few examples to help you understand what I mean: Like ricotta cheese would in lasagna, crumbled or blended tofu would work well as a filler in both sweet and savory recipes.

When it comes to saucy foods like meatloaf and Bolognese, lentils work particularly well. Continue reading to find a chapter with a variety of mouthwatering, entirely plant-based main course recipes. All in all, when this is handled perfectly, you will not even miss your non-plant based favorite meals.

Create a Support System:

Any new habit is difficult to form, but it doesn't have to be. Find some friends or family members who are willing to join you in this lifestyle. This will give you emotional support, some type of accountability, and will also help you keep motivated and focused. With these friends, you can try out new recipes, share them, or even go out to eat at establishments that serve a variety of plant-based dishes. To take it a step further and increase your knowledge and support network, you can search for local plant-based groups on social media.

What You Stand to Gain from a Plant-Based Diet is covered in Chapter 2.

The Advantages of a Plant-Based Diet

A whole food plant-based diet has the potential to reduce the symptoms of many chronic conditions, including heart disease, type 2 diabetes, arthritis, cancer, autoimmune disorders, kidney stones, inflammatory bowel diseases, and many more. Additionally, a plant-based diet is more affordable, particularly when you buy locally grown, organic foods that are in season. So let's look at the advantages of a plant-based diet.

*It Lowers Blood Pressure

Plant-based foods typically include higher amounts of potassium, which has numerous advantages including lowering blood pressure and easing anxiety and tension. Fruits, whole grains, nuts, seeds, and legumes are some foods high in potassium. On the other hand, meat has virtually no potassium.

*It brings down cholesterol

Even the saturated sources, like cacao and coconut,

do not contain cholesterol. Therefore, adopting a plant-based lifestyle will aid in lowering your body's cholesterol levels, which will minimize your risk of developing heart disease.

*Checks the Levels of Your Blood Sugar

Foods made from plants typically include a lot of fiber. This keeps you feeling fuller for longer periods of time and slows the absorption of sugar into the bloodstream. Additionally, it assists in restoring blood cortisol balance, which lessens stress.

*It Aids in the Prevention and Treatment of Chronic Diseases

Chronic diseases including cancer, obesity, and diabetes are typically quite uncommon in civilizations where the bulk of people live plant-based lifestyles. Additionally, this diet has been shown to increase the lifespan of

those who already have these chronic illnesses.

*It Promotes Weight Loss

Without using calorie limitations, eating whole plant-based foods makes it simpler to lose extra weight and keep it off while maintaining a healthier weight. This is because eating more fiber, vitamins, and minerals than you do animal fats and proteins causes weight loss to happen naturally.

What to Watch Out For If You Choose This Lifestyle

The majority of people who want to eat only plants always have a serious issue about protein.

There is this misconception that's propagated by the mainstream media backed by corporate meat producers that protein is exclusively found in meat. That's simply not true, though.

Protein is abundant in traditional staples like nuts, beans, oats, and brown rice.

Many times, calcium and other nutrients are touted as only originating from animal-based sources. The truth is that foods with high calcium content include kale, broccoli, and almonds. If calcium comes from meat, where did the animal acquire it from, ask yourself? They consume greens, so that must be the cause.

For most people who follow a plant-based diet, vitamin B12 is typically their top worry.

Everyone can typically find B12 in fortified foods, particularly cereals and plant-based milk. However, those shouldn't be relied on to receive enough of this crucial vitamin. Simply taking a liquid or sublingual vitamin B12 supplement is the best course of action to ensure that there are no problems

You can live a healthy plant-based lifestyle by eating cooked and uncooked foods that are rich in green and vibrantly colored vegetables. Your body will receive the essential minerals, vitamins, and antioxidants from these.

Chapter 3: Planning and Stocking Your Pantry

A Quick Note on Planning Your Pantry

You don't need to stress about stocking while you make the switch to a whole-food, plant-based diet. You should be able to find everything you need at your neighborhood grocery shop or farmer's market. Consider purchasing sets of clear jars to be used for food storage. This will give your pantry a neat appearance. Usually, you'll have a few shelves set aside for the storage of things like grains, nuts, beans, spices, and herbs.

Foods to Stock: Stock Your Pantry: A Plant-Based Diet's Food Guide Non-Starchy Vegetables

slender leaves (Kale, Spinach, Butter Lettuce etc.)

.Broccoli

.Zucchini

.Eggplant

.Tomatoes

*Veggies that are starchy

.potatoes of all varieties

.whole corn

.Legumes (all beans and lentils) (all beans and lentils)

.vegetable roots

.Quinoa

*Fruits

.whole fruits (avoid dried and juiced fruits)

*whole grains

.100% whole grain, oats, and brown rice

*Beverages

.Green tea, water

.Stevia-free plant-based milk

.Tea and coffee without caffeine

*Nuts

.Peanuts

.Almonds

.Cashews

.Walnuts

*Foods to Consume Sparingly

.Avocadoes

.Coconuts

.Sesame seeds

.Sunflower seeds

.Pumpkin seeds

.Dried fruit

.Added sweeteners (maple syrup, fruit juice concentrate, and natural

sugars)

.Caffeinated tea and coffee

.Alcoholic beverages

.Refined soy protein and wheat protein

*Foods to Avoid Meat

.Fish

.Poultry

.Seafood

.Red meat

.Processed meat

*Dairy

.Yogurt

.Milk

.Cheese

.Cream

.Half and half

.Buttermilk

*Added Fats

   .Liquid oils

   .Coconut oil

   .Margarine

   .Butter

*Beverages

   .Soda

   .Fruit juice

.Sports drinks

.Energy drinks

.Blended coffee and tea drinks

*Refined Flours

.All wheat flours that are not 100% whole wheat

*Vegan Replacement Foods

.Vegan "cheese" or vegan "meats" containing any oil

*Miscellaneous

.Eggs

.Candy bars

.Pastries

.Cookies

.Cakes

.Energy bars

A Few Words About Labels

Always bear in mind that the objective is not to eat a lot of items that require packaging or labeling when stocking your cupboard. It's acceptable to occasionally include that packaged food item on your list, though. These pointers will assist you in remaining alert and ensuring a safe shopping experience when this does occur.

Do Not Believe Company Claims On packaged foods, phrases like "low in fat" or "50% less sodium" are very common. They are essentially meaningless. The ingredient list and the nutrition label are what you should be paying attention to instead. It does not imply that a bag of potato chips is healthy just because it is marked as having 40% less sodium. It may still include a lot of sodium or contain a variety of other undesirable elements. The same holds true for goods with a "low-fat" designation.

Establish a Routine of Examining the Ingredient List Generally speaking, the healthier the food is, the less the ingredients it has. These foods are beneficial to your health because they frequently contain few or no additives or preservatives. It's usually a sign that a food contains a lot of sugar when the ingredients list contains a lot of words that end in "-ose." Also, look to see whether the ingredient list contains any animal products.

Chapter 4: Breakfast and Brunch Recipes

Maple Granola with Banana Whipped Topping Ingredients

2 cups of rolled oats

¼ cup of raw sunflower seeds

¼ cup of raw pumpkin seeds

¼ cup of raw unsweetened shredded dried coconut

¼ cup chopped walnuts

¼ cup raw or toasted wheat germ

1 teaspoon ground cinnamon

½ cup maple syrup

¾ cup raisins

Banana Whipped Topping, optional

For Banana Whipped Topping

8 ounces soft or firm regular tofu, drained (sprouted variety is preferred)

1 ripe banana

2 tablespoons maple syrup, plus more as needed

Instructions

i. Line a baking sheet with parchment paper and

preheat your oven to

330 degrees F.

ii. Combine oats, pumpkin seeds, walnuts, sunflower seeds, cinnamon

and wheat germ in a bowl along with maple syrup.

iii. Now in your baking sheet, spread the mixture evenly and bake

for about 20 minutes.

iv. Stir in raisins and bake for another 5 minutes until the oats aregolden.

v. Transfer to another baking sheet or tray and let it cool. You can serve it with banana toppings.

For Topping

Combine topping ingredients in a blender until smooth. Add maple syrup as desired.

Chickpea Flour Scramble Ingredients Chickpea flour batter:

½ cup of chickpea flour or use ½ cup + 1 or 2 tablespoons of more gram flour

½ cup of water

1 tablespoon of nutritional yeast

1 tablespoon of flaxseed meal

½ teaspoon of baking powder

¼ teaspoon of salt

¼ teaspoon of turmeric

¼ teaspoon or less paprika

1/8 teaspoon of Indian Sulphur black salt for the eggy flavor

Generous dash of black pepper

For Veggies:

1 teaspoon of oil divided

1 clove of garlic

¼ cup chopped onions

2 tablespoons each of asparagus green bell pepper, zucchini or other veggies.

½ green chili, chopped

2 tablespoons of chopped red bell pepper or tomato

Cilantro and black pepper for garnish

Instructions

i. Blend all the ingredients under chickpea flour batter and keep aside.

You can also use lentil batter from my lentil frittata.

ii. Heat ½ teaspoon of oil in a skillet over medium heat. Add onion and garlic and cook for about 3 minutes until translucent.

iii. Add veggies, chili and cook for another 2 mins, then add spices and greens.

iv. Cover the veggies with the chickpea flour batter and continue cooking while adding olive oil.

v. Since the mixture tends to get doughy, be sure to

scrap the bottom.Cook until the edges dry out. This should take about 5 minutes.

vi. Turn off the stove and break the food into smaller chunks then season with salt and pepper. You can garnish with cilantro if you like. Serve with toast or tacos.

*Peanut Butter and Jam Porridge Ingredients Peanut butter granola

.½ cup of rolled oats or an assortment of cereals/nuts/seeds in your pantry

.1 tablespoon peanut butter

.1 teaspoon of rice malt syrup

*Raspberry chia jam

.¼ cup raspberries

.1 tablespoon chia seeds

*Turmeric Steel Cut Oats Ingredients

.¼ teaspoon of olive oil

.½ cup of steel cut oats use certified gluten-free if needed

.1½ cup of water 2 cups for a thinner consistency

.1 cup of non-dairy milk

.1/3 teaspoon of turmeric

.½ teaspoon of cinnamon

.¼ teaspoon of cardamom

.Salt to taste

.2 tablespoons or more, of maple or other sweetener of your choice

Instructions

i. Toast oats in oil in a saucepan for a couple of minutes.

ii. Add water and milk and bring it to a boil before letting it simmer.

iii. Mix in the spices, salt, and maple and cook for about 8 minutes or until the oats are cooked to preference.

iv. Taste and adjust sweet, and flavors as desired then let it cool to thicken. You can serve warm or chilled.

v. Garnish with strawberries, dried fruit or chia seeds.

Chapter 5: Main Course Recipes

Mashed Cauliflower and Green Bean Casserole Ingredients

¾ cup of coconut milk

½ cup of nutritional yeast

1 cauliflower

Salt and pepper to taste

14 ounces of green beans, trimmed

1 onion, diced

Instructions

i. In a skillet, cook cauliflower florets in vegetable broth and some olive oil.

ii. Add in onions and beans and cook for a little longer. Transfer the mixture into a blender and add coconut milk, nutritional yeast, salt and pepper and blend until smooth.

iii. In a baking sheet, assemble green bean mix, mashed cauliflower, and toppings and bake for 15 to 20 minutes at 400 degrees F.

Enjoy.

Zucchini Noodles with Portobello Bolognese Ingredients

.3 tablespoons extra virgin olive oil, divided

.6 Portobello mushroom caps, stems, and gills removed and finely chopped

.½ cup of minced carrot

.½ cup of minced celery

.½ cup of minced yellow onion

.3 large garlic cloves, minced

.Kosher salt

.Fresh ground pepper

.1 tablespoon of tomato paste

.A 28-ounce can crushed tomatoes (I strongly recommend San Marzano)

.2 teaspoons of dried oregano

.¼ teaspoon of crushed red pepper (optional)

.½ cup fresh basil leaves, finely chopped (plus extra for serving)

.4 medium zucchin

Instructions

i. Sauté garlic, mushrooms, celery, and carrots in olive oil in a pan.

Season with salt and pepper as desired. Continue cooking until vegetables are soft.

ii. Stir in some tomato paste and cook for a couple of minutes before adding crushed tomatoes, oregano, red pepper, and basil.

iii. Let it simmer for 10 to 15 minutes until the sauce thickens.

iv. As the sauce simmers, use an appropriate blade to make spiral zucchini.

v. Sauté the zucchini noodles in a separate saucepan for a couple of minutes and season as desired.

vi. Top with a generous amount of Bolognese and garnish with freshly chopped basil and serve immediately.

Chapter 6: Dessert and Treats Recipes

Cream Decorated Truffles Ingredients For the truffles:

2 tablespoons of organic raw cacao

½ cup of organic raw zucchini

½ cup of rolled oats

¼ cup Medjool dates or raisins

For the cream:

½ cup cashews

½ teaspoons of alcohol-free vanilla extract

2 Medjool dates, pitted

For decorating:

1 tablespoon filtered water

½ tsp. organic raw cacao

Instructions

i. Combine truffle ingredients in a blender until fully-fused.

ii. Using wet hands form the mixture into small balls and set aside.

iii. Combine cream ingredients in a blender until smooth then spread it over some of the truffles.

iv. Add two small pea size quantities of cream for the mummies' eyeballs for the remaining truffles.

v. Mix water and cacao in a small bowl and use a toothpick to make drops of the mixture onto the truffles. Enjoy.

Raw Orange Chocolate Pudding Ingredients

1 vanilla bean, seeds scraped out (or 1 ½ tsp pure vanilla extract)

A cup of peeled, pitted, and roughly chopped ripe avocado

1 cup pitted dates

1/3 cup raw or regular cocoa powder

1 teaspoon of orange zest

½ cup of freshly squeezed orange juice

1/8 teaspoon of sea salt

Instructions

i. Combine all ingredients in a food processor and puree until smooth.

ii. You can thin the puree by adding more orange juice, or a splash of nut milk or water.

iii. Serve or store in the refrigerator.

Mango Chia Seed Pudding Ingredients

2 cups of coconut milk

½ cup of chia seeds

1 teaspoon of vanilla (powder or extract)

¼ teaspoon of cardamom

1 medium sized mango

3 tablespoons of coconut nectar or 2 tablespoons of date paste

Instructions

i. Mix chia seeds with coconut milk, coconut nectar, vanilla, and cardamom in a bowl and refrigerate up to overnight.

ii. Slice the mango up into pieces and puree in a blender.

iii. Serve accordingly – mix together or serve in layers and enjoy!

Berry Basil Popsicles Ingredients

1½ cup of sliced strawberries

1 cup of mixed berries (I used raspberry, red currant, and

blueberry)

10 to 20 fresh basil leaves

A tablespoon of lemon juice

1 to 3 tablespoons of maple syrup (optional

Instructions

i. Combine all ingredients in a blender until smooth.

ii. Pour the mixture into Popsicle molds and insert Popsicle sticks.

Freeze overnight. Enjoy!

Red Velvet Cake Smoothie Ingredients

2 ripe bananas, peeled

½ medium beet, scrubbed and roughly chopped

½ cup of walnut pieces

4 to 6 pitted dates, depending on how sweet you want it

1 cup fresh packed spinach

¼ cup of unsweetened cocoa powder

1 teaspoon of pure vanilla extract

1½ cups of non-dairy milk such as almond, rice, or

coconut

2 cups of ice

Optional Garnish:

Finely chopped dark chocolate

Finely chopped walnuts

Coconut flakes

Instructions

i. Combine all ingredients in a blender until a smoothie consistency is achieved.

ii. Garnish as desired and serve!

Vegan Butter Coffee Ingredients

A cup high quality brewed coffee

A tablespoon of coconut butter

A tablespoon of plant-based milk of your choice

Optional add-ins:

1 teaspoon of MCT oil

1 teaspoon of cinnamon

1 teaspoon of vanilla powder

1 teaspoon of coconut milk powder (instead of the plant milk)

Instructions

i. Brew your coffee – either a French press or automatic coffee maker using high-quality coffee.

ii. Add a cup of coffee in a blender along with coconut butter and other add-ins and blend until foamy.

iii. Pour in a mug and top with foamed plant milk or dust with cinnamon.

Lemon Lime Lavender Smoothie Ingredients

1½ cups of plant yogurt

3 tablespoons of lemon juice

4 tablespoons of lime juice

A drop of lavender extract, culinary OR ½ teaspoon of culinary lavender buds¼ cup of ice cubes

½ teaspoon of turmeric (or more to achieve desired color)

¼ cup of shavings from fresh organic lemons and limes

Instructions

i. Combine all the ingredients in a blender and serve chilled with citrus shavings and lavender buds on top for a strong scent as you spoon!

ii. Add some plant-based milk to thin mixture.

Apple Spinach Protein Smoothie Ingredients

1 large organic apple

3 to 4 cups of organic spinach

A tablespoon of organic almond butter

1 scoop (or packet) Vega Sport vanilla protein powder

1 cup of unsweetened original almond milk

4 to 5 ice cubes

Instructions

i. Add all the ingredients except spinach to a blender and process until smooth.

ii. Add spinach in batches, blending a handful at a time until it is all incorporated.

iii. Pour into a glass and enjoy!

Herby Crust Asparagus Spears Ingredients

1 bunch of asparagus

2 tablespoons of hemp seeds

¼ cup of nutritional yeast

1 teaspoon of garlic powder or 3 garlic cloves, minced

1/8 teaspoon of ground pepper

Pinch of paprika

¼ cup of whole wheat breadcrumbs

Juice of ½ a lemon

Instructions

i. Preheat the oven to 350°F.

ii. Wash the asparagus and remove the white bottom end.

iii. Transfer hemp seeds to a small bowl and mix in the nutritional yeast, garlic, pepper, paprika, and breadcrumbs. Stir and set aside.

iv. In a baking dish, place the asparagus spears side by side sprinkle over hemp mixture.

v. Bake for 20 to 30 minutes to achieve crispy asparagus.

vi. Serve and sprinkle with some lemon juice.

Green Pea Guacamole Ingredients

2 cups of frozen green peas, thawed

1 teaspoon crushed garlic

¼ cup of fresh lime juice

½ teaspoon of ground cumin

1 tomato, chopped

4 green onions, chopped

½ cup of chopped fresh cilantro

⅛ of a teaspoon of hot sauce

Sea salt to taste

Instructions

i. Blend the peas, garlic, lime juice, and cumin in a food processor until smooth.

ii. Stir in the tomato, green onion, cilantro, and hot sauce and transfer into a bowl. Season as desired.

iii. Cover and refrigerate for half an hour before serving.

Mint Chip Energy Bites Ingredients

1/8 teaspoon peppermint extract

Pinch of fine sea salt

2 tablespoons mini chocolate chips

10 Medjool dates, pitted

½ cup of coconut flakes

½ cup of chopped walnuts

¼ cup of cocoa powder

Instructions

i. Add dates to your food processor and process until broken up into pea-sized bits.

ii. Add in coconut flakes, walnuts, cocoa powder, peppermint extract,and a pinch of salt and continue processing until it is well combined into a large ball.

iii. Roll the mixture into roughly 1-inch balls and freeze for 20 minutes then transfer to refrigerator.

No-Bake Brownie Energy Bites Ingredients Dry Ingredients:

½ cup gluten-free oat flour

½ cup unsweetened cocoa powder

¼ cup ground flaxseed

½ cup vegan chocolate chips

Wet Ingredients:

¾ cup natural, unsalted creamy almond butter

¼ cup pure maple syrup

1 teaspoon pure vanilla extract

Instructions

i. In a large bowl, mix together all of the dry ingredients: oat flour,cocoa powder, flaxseed and chocolate chips.

ii. Add vanilla, maple syrup and almond butter whilst stirring and folding using a spatula.

iii. Using a cookie scoop, scoop and drop a ball into your hands.

Roll and press into bites. Enjoy!

Potato Pancakes Ingredients

2 russet potatoes, grated

1 large zucchini, grated

½ yellow onion, grated

½ cup of oat flour

A teaspoon of baking powder

½ teaspoon of freshly ground black pepper

Instructions

i. Preheat oven to 420 degrees. Cover two sheet pans with parchment paper.

ii. Spread half of the grated vegetables on a clean kitchen towel, then roll and wring the towel to draw out the excess moisture.

iii. Transfer to a large mixing bowl. Repeat with the remaining vegetables.

iv. In a small bowl, combine the oat flour, baking powder, and pepper and add to the vegetable bowl, and mix well, using your hands to evenly distribute the flour and baking powder.

v. Scoop some of the potato mixture, and hand-shape it into a semi tight ball. Flatten with your palms, and place the pancake onto the prepared pan. Repeat with the remaining mix, spacing the pancakes appropriately.

vi. Bake for no more than 15 minutes. Flip and bake for another 10 or

so minutes. Top with the condiment of your choice.

BONUS: Make Your Plant-Based Lifestyle a Success

Key Pillars Going Forward

Water

Water contains no calories, fat, or cholesterol and is low in sodium. It is nature's appetite suppressant, and it helps the body to metabolize fat thereby helping you lose weight.

Fiber

There are a slew of health benefits that come with consuming lots of dietary fiber. They include: Normalizing bowel movements and maintaining bowel health Lower blood cholesterol levels Helps control blood sugar levels

Promote healthier gut bacteria Reduce risk of certain cancers

Rest and Sleep

Going forward, adequate rest and sleep will become a major pillar in your quest to lead a healthy lifestyle. The importance of sleep and rest cannot be overstated.

Among its numerous benefits include: Appetite regulation Reducing your calorie intake Increases your resting metabolism Prevents insulin resistance

Provide you with energy for physical activity

Positive Mindset

A positive mindset can help you maintain your plant-based diet and realize your health and fitness goals. Seeing as this requires patience and commitment, having a positive outlook and approach is going to help you: stay motivated,focus on the positive aspects of your diet and overcome emotions during your low moments.

Physical Activity

The health benefits of regular exercise and physical activity are hard to ignore.

Exercising regularly will help you: Control weight Fight off health conditions and diseases Improve your mood Boost your energy levels

Promote better sleep

Conclusion

I think you now see the advantages of a plant-based diet and lifestyle. I hope this book has all the answers you were looking for regarding this type of dieting so you can start putting it to use. You don't have to completely give up animal products if you are still on the fence about it. The key message here is to prioritize eating plant-based meals while you take modest steps toward switching to a fully plant-based lifestyle. You'll soon become aware of how much better, stronger, and healthier both your body and mind feel. Before you can cure your diet, you must first fix your health!

I would be eternally grateful if you could post a review on Amazon if you liked learning about the plant-based diet. The best way to assist your other readers in discovering excellent books is to provide reviews, so do so!